AWAKENINGS

BY EMBROSEWYN TAZKUVEL

Celestine Light Magick Series

ANGELS OF MIRACLES AND MANIFESTATION
144 Names, Sigils and Stewardships to Call the Magickal Angels of Celestine Light

WORDS OF POWER AND TRANSFORMATION
101+ Magickal Words and Sigils of Celestine Light to Manifest Your Desires

CELESTINE LIGHT MAGICKAL SIGILS OF HEAVEN & EARTH

Secret Earth Series

INCEPTION *(BOOK 1)*
DESTINY *(BOOK 2)*

Psychic Awakening Series

CLAIRVOYANCE
TELEKINESIS
DREAMS

AURAS
How to See, Feel and Know

SOUL MATE AURAS
How Find Your Soul Mate & "Happily Ever After"

UNLEASH YOUR PSYCHIC POWERS

PSYCHIC SELF DEFENSE

LOVE YOURSELF
Secret Key To Transforming Your Life

22 STEPS TO THE LIGHT OF YOUR SOUL

ORACLES OF CELESTINE LIGHT
Complete Trilogy of Genesis, Nexus & Vivus

Published by Kaleidoscope Productions
1467 Siskiyou Boulevard, #9; Ashland, OR 97520
www.kaleidoscope-publications.com
ISBN 978-0-938001-05-8

Book layout and design by Sumara Elan Love
www.3wizardz.com

AWAKENINGS

How to Awaken Someone from a Coma

Embrosewyn Tazkuvel
and Philos

TABLE OF CONTENTS

INTRODUCTION

Dealing with a loved one in a coma is always a heart-rending experience for the family members at their bedside. Not only do they have to cope with the daily anguish of seeing their beloved spouse, parent, child or friend completely unconscious and unresponsive, they also have to somehow continue to do all the daily tasks necessary to keep their own lives and their families functioning; often without the aid of adequate insurance and with a big hole left in the budget from the lost income of the loved one in a coma.

If you are reading this book now, it is likely you or someone close to you has a loved one currently in a coma. Let me admonish you, do not despair. As you read on you will find there is a lot more hope than you would often be led to believe by many doctors and the traditional medical establishment. Most people do come out of comas, many fairly quickly. An astounding number are misdiagnosed. Even those who have been in unresponsive comas for years can reawaken. It's not a wishful dream- there are many documented cases. In the final chapter of this book you will discover the powerful new treatments revealed by Filos. Even if you have been told to give up all hope, let it stir again in your heart. Because there is hope, even great hope, to bring back many of those thought to be lost.

Chapter I

WHAT IS A COMA?

When something occurs that damages or severely shocks the brain, the victim may fall into a coma. This is a very serious condition where the brain shuts down, often almost completely, making the person unable to respond to any stimulus or nearby activity. In the worst cases, the victim cannot even breathe on their own, and require the use of a mechanical ventilator to keep them alive.

Accidents are common causes of comas, especially car accidents, but also workplace accidents and even accidents at home. Comas can also be caused from many other sources including, seizures, diabetic insulin imbalances, infections in the brain or affecting the brain, prolonged lack of oxygen such as when a person has been submerged under water, deprivation of glucose, strokes, drug overdoses, profound hypothyroidism and heart attacks.

Various poisons can also directly affect the brain, both those taken in by the body and those created inside the body when certain organs like the kidneys or liver malfunction or cease functioning properly due to diseases like alcoholism. In this regard even seemingly harmless ingestions can ultimately lead to a coma. There have been multiple instances of a victim unintentionally overdosing on Acetaminophen, causing their liver to fail and within a few days they fall into a hepatic coma.

In cases of head injuries, if they are minor the brain may be knocked out of whack for a bit, including a period of unconsciousness, but usually after a short period of minutes or hours, days at the most, it restarts itself with normal function. In cases of severe brain injury, additional fluids, most often blood, frequently begin building in the brain (edema). Injury alone, without bleeding in the brain, can still cause edema. As the brain is completely encased in a solid bone skull there is no room for any additional fluid buildup or swelling. This increased pressure, if not stopped or relieved, often leads to a longer-term coma and additional physical damage to the brain. Bleeding within the brain can also be caused from non-injuries, such as high blood pressure that rises to a point that blood veins in the brain cannot withstand the pressure and begin to leak.

Thyroid problems are fairly common in the general population and this too can lead to a coma. The thyroid is the bodies' thermostat and regulates the speed at which the body operates. If the thyroid function diminishes because of a drop in thyroid hormone levels, over time hypothyroidism can result and a myxdema coma can occur.

The initial outlook for someone in a coma depends a great deal on the cause of the comatose state. Many comas are short in duration and the initial diagnosis may show something as simple as hypoglycemic low blood sugar and offer a quick resolution by correcting the sugar imbalance.

Coma patients, especially those in long-term comas, require 24 hour intensive care. As they can do nothing for themselves, they require doctors and nurses to insure they get needed fluids and medicines, often intravenously, as well as nutrition which is often through a feeding tube leading directly to their stomach. They also need frequent turning of their body to prevent bedsores, as well as regular emptying and maintaining of all the apparatus required for processing their bodily waste.

Although it is certain that some unfortunate brain-injured people fall into irreversible comas, incidence after incidence have proven that many victims are able to hear everything being said around them and desire to respond. But the lack of function in their brains leaves them trapped in their own body, unable to acknowledge loved ones by voice or even the blink of an eye or the twitch of a finger. Yet case after case has proven that many are still cognizant, and frustrated that they cannot communicate their sentience by voice or even the tiniest movement of their body, even though inside they may be crying out for help, pleading, "Hey I'm alive, I'm still here, don't leave me", or even more chilling, "don't kill me."

Seeing a loved one in a coma can be a frightening and frustrating situation for those closest to them. But there is and should be a lot of hope because victims do come out of comas, often fairly quickly and the actions, words and expressions of hope by loved ones can certainly speed the process in many cases.

Most comatose patients will awaken from their coma in just a few weeks. But unlike on TV shows and movies they usually don't instantly come back with their full abilities as if they had just been asleep. Though some of them are able to return to their normal activities, including work, many will require additional months or even years of rehabilitation. Initially, they will often feel confused and will respond slowly to words and actions happening around them. But over time, with love and effort most can have a full or near full recovery.

What degree of rehabilitation will be necessary, how long it will take and whether the formerly comatose victim will be able to return to the same level of normal function they had prior to their coma, will depend upon how much damage was done to the brain and the type and length of the rehabilitation. Occasionally, someone will come out of a coma like nothing ever happened, ready to resume their normal life. But more often, the need to relearn things as simple as eating with a utensil, walking and speaking. Loved ones can be a tremendous boon to recovery by exhibiting a lot of love, giving never-failing support and positive encouragement, and maintaining calm, harmonious patience.

Chapter II

GLASCOW COMA SCALE

The Glasgow Coma Scale, which goes by its acronym GCS, was developed by two neurosurgery professors at the University of Glascow in 1974. It is used to access the level of consciousness of a patient after a head injury, and is now widely used by EMT's, EMS's, doctors and in hospital Intensive Care wards for all types of injuries that may affect consciousness.

The lowest possible score is 3, indicating a victim in a deep coma. The highest score of 15 is indicative of a fully conscious and aware person.

The GSC was developed as a simple way for doctors and other health care professionals to quickly be able to access the level of consciousness of a brain-injured patient in an initial evaluation by observing their eye movements, speech ability, and physical reactions to stimuli. It is also frequently used to access the level of a patient's progress in recovering from a brain injury.

When the GCS score is documented; the deeper the coma, the lower the score. Please appreciate that a person with a "normal" GCS of 15 effectively can still be in a coma. Once the initial screening physical examination is complete, a more detailed exam will likely occur to include the lungs, the heart, and the abdomen. Repeated neurologic assessment is key to monitoring the status of the patient and decides if the coma is lightening or getting worse.

When a victim of an accident, injury or some other malady, exhibiting a comatose state, is brought to a hospital emergency ward, the first priority of a hospital staff is to stabilize the patients' vital signs. After stabilization, if the patient remains in an unconscious state, a thorough physical from head to toe and a complete neurological assessment will likely ensue. This will probably include blood tests, an examination of facial movements, eyes, pupils, reactions to physical stimulations, tendon reflexes and other spinal cord tests to determine the degree of function. A CT scan of the head is also often required. Special attention is paid to the neurological exam as a lack of response can indicate multiple possibilities including a stroke or bleeding inside the skull, especially if only one side of the body is affected. The decision as to what tests are initially performed will depend upon the initial assessment of the likely cause of the comatose state. After the initial assessment, doctors will continue to monitor and test the patient to determine if the comatose state is deepening or improving.

Doctors also use additional cognitive tests to assess the depth of a coma and the level of consciousness, including the Rancho Los Amigos Scale (RLAS) which is commonly used to determine the progress of recovery from traumatic brain injuries.

Chapter III

OVER 40% WRONG DIAGNOSIS!

If there is anything that stands like a beacon on a hill to give the family of coma victims hope, it is the fact that according to medical studies over 40% of the diagnosis given about comatose patients are wrong! The traditional medical community is flustered and flabbergasted when patients that have been solemnly declared to be in unrecoverable, permanent vegetative states, all of a sudden awaken, conscious and cognizant!

Here's just one of many examples:

In December of 1979, Sgt. David Mack of the Minneapolis Police Department, along with eight other officers battered their way through a door of a suspect's house in search of stolen property. The resident unleashed a hail of bullets at the charging police. Sgt. Mack was shot in the neck and abdomen. He stopped breathing and lapsed into a coma, likely from the lack of oxygen to his brain. Six months later, one of his neurologists, Dr. Ronald E. Cranford, solemnly announced that, "Sergeant Mack will never regain cognitive, sapient functioning. He will never be aware of his condition nor resume any degree of meaningful voluntary conscious interaction with his family or friends."

Almost two years after the shooting, in October of 1981, doctors were stunned to discover that Sgt. Mack was conscious and even more startled to realize that his intellect was intact.

Dr. Cranford, contritely admitted the misdiagnose and called into question similar diagnosis that is often applied to other comatose patients, saying, "The fact that Mack awoke calls into question the way we assess these cases. It introduces an element of uncertainty into a situation that was very difficult to begin with."

This admission is even more surprising coming from Dr. Cranford who is a well-known proponent of euthanasia. He calls himself "Dr. Humane Death" and is a popular expert witness in right-to-die trials across the United States.

An article in Medical News, June 20th, 2007, confirmed that, " ...around 40% of patients were wrongly diagnosed as in a vegetative state..." and cautioned, "New studies underline the importance of extreme caution in any decision to limit the life chances of patients during the acute phase of a vegetative state."

At a medical conference of the European Neurological Society held in Greece, June 1st through June 20th that same year, doctors addressing the assembly stated that a "significant portion" of coma patients in intensive care may just be in a transitory state, with a wide range of possible recovery scenarios."

In a paper published by K. Andrews, L. Murphy, R. Munday and C. Underwood, the results of their study of 40 coma patients in a rehabilitation unit, admitted between 1992 and 1995, concluded that "43% were considered misdiagnosed, seven of these had been presumed to be vegetative for longer than one year, including three for over four years."

Even patients that have been in assumed comas for several years have astonished their doctors when they not only suddenly awaken, but do so with their intellect and personality intact. One such case occurred in March of 2007, when Christa Lilly, 49, who suffered a cardiac arrest in November 2000, and who had been being cared for since then at home by her mother, awakened for three days before relapsing, readily talking with her family members and excitedly asking to eat some of her favorite foods.

Christa's mother had told the doctors that her daughter was waking from time to time and could speak to her normally, but it was assumed it was a fantasy of the mothers rather than a reality. But when Christa awakened and remained awake for three days her doctors all had time to come and witness her transformation for themselves. One her doctors, Randall Bjork who had been skeptical of the mothers previous reports of Christa's awakening, said he was now a believer, even if he didn't understand how it could occur, admitting, "This is all mystical and I can't explain it." He spoke about the degree of her cognizance, recounting, "She was smiling and grinning and told my staff she wanted to go to a club, even doing a little chair dance in her wheelchair." Realizing the profound implications of Christa's awakening, Dr. Bjork added, "We may have to rethink these people that have been called vegetative in nursing homes who may have some awareness of their horrible circumstances," said Dr. Bjork. "It goes against the grain of what we thought."

Chapter IV

A BARBARIC WAY TO LET SOMEONE DIE

Like many people in the United States and many countries abroad, I kept close watch on the Terry Shiavo drama as it developed over the years and finally culminated in her death in March of 2005 by starvation and dehydration after her feeding tubes were removed. Regardless of whether you thought Terry Shiavo's life should have been ended or not, my question for all is to consider, how can we accept ending anyone's life in the dehumanizing manner of death by slow starvation and dehydration?

Honestly, I was aghast that ending someone's life in this manner could be considered humane by anyone. I kept remembering my cat afflicted by a terminal disease that had completely debilitated him. When we accepted that he was suffering and in pain, that there was no hope for recovery, no hope for any fulfillment in his life, we took him to the vet and the vet gave him a shot to painlessly and quickly end his life. We held him in our hands as a family as the shot was administered so his last moments would be full of all of our love and affection. In a matter of seconds after the injection he closed his eyes for the last time and in less than a minute he was gone from this life, painlessly, quickly, and surrounded by the love and embrace of all of his family.

As Terry Shiavo was put into her final death spiral, with

the removal of her feeding tubes, she was left to die slowly of starvation and dehydration in an ordeal that even stunned many doctors by taking fourteen days before she finally perished. And through every day of her ordeal I kept thinking of my cat, and the many thousands of other cats, dogs, horses and even birds that are loved by families all over the world who are painlessly and quickly "put to sleep" when it is judged by their loved ones that they are suffering too much. I kept asking myself over and over, how can it be that we as a human(e) race are OK to put our animals "to sleep" to end their suffering, but when it comes to human members of our family that we in any way, religious or otherwise, can justify ending their lives in a slow torture of no food or water? Why don't the human members of our family deserve the same consideration, love and compassion as our animals?

It is likely that 99.9% of the people who consider euthanasia by starvation and dehydration as a way of ending the life of one of their loved ones, actually have no idea what that entails. Elaborating on what the effects would be when Terry Shiavo's feeding tubes were removed, constitutional attorney and author John W. Whitehead gave a vivid description of what would follow. "The first effects of starvation and dehydration when the feeding tube is removed include the mouth drying out and the tongue becoming swollen and cracked. When a person is slowly killed in this way, the lips become parched and cracked, and a thick coating may begin to cake the mouth and lips. The eyes will sink back into the skull, while the cheeks will hollow. The lining of the nose will begin to crack, too, possibly causing nosebleeds. The skin will turn dry and scaly and hang loose on the bones. Urine decreases, becoming highly concentrated, and eventually stops completely; then the stomach lining dries out, causing vomiting and dry heaves. Brain cells dry out too, causing convulsions. The respiratory tract dries out and thick secretions develop, which may plug the lungs and airways. Eventually, after the body suffers all these effects, all the major organs fail, including the lungs, heart and brain."

An anonymous commenter on a forum I read while researching this book put this issue into sharp perspective noting, "It's sad that we live in a world where we show mercy to death row inmates, but to those whom are sick we show no mercy. In Colorado if you were to starve a pet you would go to jail for a minimum of 10 years. What gives?"

Regardless of what side of the fence you stand on the issue of euthanasia of patients labeled in a "persistent vegetative state" by some doctors, I would beg you to consider the inhumanity of death by starvation and dehydration, which especially in the case of a defenseless coma patient, is the final and most cruel indignity.

Some will vehemently disagree that Terry Shiavo or any other patient whose life is so ended, suffered at all. Denying the evidence of the frighteningly deteriorating body before them, they'll argue that she feels no pain, and does not suffer in any way. Even if that was true, which many in the medical and ethical community would dispute, if you have already sentenced her to die, why dehumanize her by removing her food and hydration and allowing her body to slowly shrivel as the water diminishes in every cell? Why not just give her a lethal injection and let her die with at least the dignity of her body's appearance intact?

Chapter V

HOPE IN ALTERNATIVE TREATMENTS

Given the acknowledged high number of misdiagnosis and the not infrequent cases of supposedly brain-dead patients regaining consciousness, cognizance and mobility, many people and doctors are calling into question long-held assumptions and practices regarding patients in persistent vegetative states. In the past it was assumed if a comatose brain did not restart in a fairly short period of time, it was an almost sure indicator that it never would. Once so diagnosed, there was little incentive to continue to use limited resources to maintain the life of "hopeless" cases.

As the case of Sgt. Mack and many other coma patients that have reawakened attest, their verdict of inescapable internal prison and ultimate organ failure and death has been wrong.

The very definition of what is and is not "brain dead" is now being seriously debated. Thirty-one states, including Washington D.C. have legally enshrined that death is official when the brain is dead. The problem that now is obvious is that many diagnosis of a brain death are incorrect and even far off the mark, given the many unexpected and unexplained recoveries from long-term comas.

In the last decade the debate has been stoked by the success of a range of alternative treatments. Although the methods vary, they share a common belief and faith in the restorative powers of the brain and the ability of most comatose patients to get better.

For the first time, some hospitals are making extensive, long-term nursing care available. In the past many comatose patients were just allowed to slowly deteriorate with minimal care and no effort toward rehabilitation. In clinics and other institutions with a focus on coma patient recovery, patients are given intense external stimulation such as ice cubes on their bare skin or loud noises crashing beside them in attempts to reactivate their mind. Even some forms of electro-stimulation have been utilized. Because there are no standardized procedures for treating coma patients focused on rehabilitation, and the patients have most often been written off as "incurable," the medical community has not interfered with the many alternative treatments being used.

However, the issue of how to properly treat comatose patients is a more pressing one. Because of advances in emergency room trauma care and intensive-care technology, including massive doses of barbiturates to control pressure in the brain, 50 percent more brain injured patients survive than did just 20 years ago.

In light of the high number of misdiagnosis and the breakthrough advances in both trauma care and surprising reawakening of some coma victims, now more than ever, the question of whether a patient is truly brain-dead (the most accepted definition of clinically dead) with their body just kept functioning by machines, or is someone that might exhibit no cortex brain activity but somehow still be alive and capable of reawakening, is far more than just a simple moral or ethical judgment. The accepted medical science itself has been thrown into disarray as recent awakenings have proven past premises incorrect.

It is widely agreed that if the brain stem is destroyed the rest of the brain will soon die. The problem has arisen in the past that patients with intact brain stems but a non-functioning cortex, the seat of higher functions such as thoughts and emotions, have been condemned to death at worst, or an ignoring of their rehabilitative needs at best, by the what is obviously in many cases a false premise that the cortex cannot be reignited.

Tony Conigliaro, a former Boston Red Sox star, is one example of the success of alternative treatments and the power of the human brain to regenerate and restore lost function. After suffering a massive heart attack that deprived his brain of oxygen for over 10 minutes he went into a deep coma with a prognosis of little to no chance of recovery. His father insisted his son be given alternative treatments and he was willing to try many. Tony was given a derivative of wheat germ oil by a nutritionist, low-voltage electrical treatments by an osteopath, energy gateway openings by an acupuncturist and auric treatments by a Russian psychic. Though the medical professionals scoffed at all these unorthodox treatments, to their utter surprise and inability to explain, Tony emerged from his coma. His first words were, "Hi, Mom. Hi, Dad."

One facility that has intentionally created a space to treat patients in a persistent vegetative state with alternative therapies is the Greenery, a 200-bed nursing home in Boston. They have on average 40 patients in the coma ward with cognitive levels so unregisterable that there are few other if any facilities in the country that could take them for therapy.

At the Greenery they are housed in bright colored rooms full of sunlight. Nurses, along with physical and occupational therapists and assistants put their patients through a rigorous daily regimen. They carry on regular conversations with them as if they were hearing, understanding and answering. They are continually being touched and are given regular exercise, even if it is all done by the therapist manipulating their limbs. Twice during the day they are given heightened stimulation where they are exposed to bells, whistles, ice water, peanut butter and other strong sensory inputs. Brightly colored balls, soap bubbles and other eye-catching items are moved in front of their eyes to induce them to track the objects.

Then there's Dr. Mihai D. Dimancescu, a Long Island, New York, neurosurgeon, who practices structured stimulation, which includes many sensory exercises, for up to 16 hours a day, every day, oftentimes for months. Dr. Dimancescu focuses on a key but little known activity of the brain known as "reticular activating formation." This is the brain mechanism that is continually monitoring stimuli from the outside world, 24 hours a day, awake or asleep. It is a sentinel to alert the person to any stimuli they encounter, prompting the person to either react or ignore, whether the sound is the wind whistling through the trees or an alarm bell clanging nearby.

Dr. Dimancescu's regime dictates daily stimuli many times during the day including extremely bright lights turned on and off multiple times, ammonia held under the nose for up to 5 seconds, two blocks of wood loudly smashed together, painful pressure applied to each fingernail for 5 seconds, and physical stimulation to each joint in the neck, shoulders, wrists, elbows, fingers, hips, knees and ankles. Each may be put through up to 200 manipulations a day.

Dr. Dimancescu claims he has a 92% success rate although his peers in the medical establishment remain doubtful until he publishes his results officially. He says his success comes from a simple formula, "knock on the door as hard as you can, as often as you can, for as long as you can."

Chapter VI

RECENT MEDICAL BREAKTHROUGH

What if a coma patient could simply take a small pill and within minutes awaken from their coma? Is this a fantasy of family members refusing to give up hope or reality of the most amazing magnitude? Believe it or not, in many cases lending great hope for future treatment of victims in a vegetative state, this is a reality. In recent years, on three different continents, patients in deep, persistent vegetative states, including those that had been labeled "brain-damaged vegetables," have resoundingly and suddenly awakened with full cognizance, by taking a commonly used sleeping pill! And the doctor who made this accidental discovery, along with many others who work with coma patients around the world, were initially uncomprehending and continue to be stunned that this has occurred.

The mystery of the astounding awakenings from a simple sleeping pill began in 1994 at the Ikaya Tinivorster Rehabilitation Center in South Africa. Louis Viljoen, a 24 year old switchboard operator, received severe, coma-inducing head injuries when he was hit by a truck while riding his bike in a suburb of Johannesburg. He fell into a deep coma and remained completely unresponsive for five years. His mother, Sienie Engelbrecht visited him every day, despite being told by the doctors that her son had no hope of recovery and that they expected him to die. Yet she had no indication that any other outcome was possible. She explained, "His eyes were open but there was nothing there. I visited him every day for five years and we would speak to him but there was no recognition, no communication, nothing."

One of the people who looked in on Louis was the hospital ward sister, Lucy Hughes. After observing repeated involuntary spasms in Louis's left arm, which caused him to tear his mattress, she worried that he might be experiencing internal discomfort and suggested to Louis's mother that she ask his doctor to prescribe a sedative. Dr. Wally Nel subsequently prescribed Stilnox; the brand name in South Africa for the sleeping pill Zolpidem, assuming it would put Louis into a deep sleep. His mother Sienie recounted what happened next. "I crushed it up and gave it to him in a bottle with a soft drink. He couldn't swallow properly then, but I helped him and sat at his bedside. After about 25 minutes, I heard him making a sound like "mmm." He hadn't made a sound for five years. Then he turned his head in my direction. I said, "Louis, can you hear me?" And he said, "Yes." I said, "Say hello, Louis," and he said, "Hello, mummy." I couldn't believe it. I just cried and cried."

Lucy Hughes and other staff members were excitedly called over and they gathered around Louis in stunned amazement. Hughes recalled, "Sienie told me he was talking and I said he couldn't be - it wasn't possible. Then I heard him. His mother was speechless and so were we. It was a very emotional moment."

Louis continues to receive a dose of Zolpidem every day and has been since his initial awakening in 1999. Because

Zolpidem is a drug, to limit possible side-effects he can't receive it every time he slips out of consciousness. But the long-term beneficial effects are undeniable. Though the effects of the drug are supposed to end after a little over 2 hours in his body, Louis continues to improve in almost every measurable category. It's as if the engine of the brain has been switched back on. Though he was once referred to as "a cabbage" by a thoughtless doctor, today Louis greets visitors with a mischievous grin and not uncommonly a complicated four-move street handshake.

One investigator had the opportunity to speak with Louis and witness his daily transformation. Here is his account: "I see Louis before his daily medication, yet he is conscious where once he would have been comatose. Almost blind because of a separate and deteriorating condition, there is a droop to one side of his mouth and brow because of brain damage. His right arm is twisted awkwardly into his side.

Louis is given a pill, and I watch. It is 8.30am. After nine minutes the grey pallor disappears and his face flushes. He starts smiling and laughing. After 10 minutes he begins asking questions. His speech is impaired because of the brain damage and the need, several years ago, to remove all his teeth, but I can understand him. A couple of minutes later, his right arm becomes less contorted and the facial drooping lessens. After 15 minutes he reaches out to hug Sienie. He pulls off her wedding ring and asks what it is. "It's a suffer-ring," she jokes. And he says, "Well, if you're suffering, you should make a plan!" The banter continues and he remembers conversations from the previous day and adds to them.

"Louis," I ask, "do you feel any change in awareness before and after the pill?" "No," he says, "None whatsoever." Whatever is happening, he feels the same. "How do you know this is your mother?" I ask, referring to Sienie. Remember, Louis cannot see. He says: "Because I recognize her voice and I know she loves me."

Louis's doctor, Wally Nel continues to be as fulfilled and amazed as everyone else at the remarkable and immediate transformation that occurs in Louis after taking just one little pill. "Something strange and wonderful is happening here, and we have to get to the bottom of it," he says. "Since Louis, I have treated more than 150 brain-damaged patients with Zolpidem and have seen improvements in about 60% of them. It's remarkable."

Louis reaction soon proved that it was not some anomalous fluke. Word quickly spread in the coma community in South Africa and the results began to be replicated with other patients.

Following a horrible car crash Riaan Bolton lay motionless for three years. His unwavering eyes wide open but reacting to nothing they were looking at. An enthusiastic cricketer and rugby player, the 23 year old was studying to become an industrial engineer. Doctors told his mother Johanna that her son would never again be able to see, speak or hear. She was asked if she wanted to let him die as there was no hope.

"One specialist said he had a 5% chance of recovering, another said he had no chance whatsoever of regaining consciousness," says his mother, Johanna. She and her husband Tinus refused to let Riaan die. They took him home, converted their garage into a mini-convalescent center and spent about £1,000 a month on round-the-clock care. Despite all their efforts they saw no awareness or improvement in their son's condition.

Hearing about the success of Dr. Nel, they asked their doctor, Clive Holroyd to contact him, and Riaan soon received his first dose of Zolpidem. Tinus recounted what happened next. "There was no movement, no recognition, just nothing," says Tinus. "Then we gave him the pill and we noticed him moving the fingers in his left hand and touching them against each other. His eyes went big and he began looking from left to right. The doctor started asking Riaan questions. He said, "Look at me, Riaan" and Riaan looked straight at him and focused on his face. Then the doctor asked him to move his hand and he moved it. And then he lifted his head from the pillow and began looking around. I couldn't believe it."

"It has given us hope," says Johanna. "To have communication with him again, to know he becomes aware of us and to tell him we love him - knowing he can hear us - is simply beyond belief. It has been a very moving experience."

Dr. Holroyd remains perplexed. "There is a measurement of the depths of coma called the Glasgow scale, with three being the worst and 15 being normal," he says. "Riaan was six, but within 10 minutes of taking the pill he is up to nine. It's simply unbelievable. And the mind-boggling thing about this is that it's done with a sleeping pill. Some time ago, Riaan had a cardiac arrest and it was a difficult call as to whether or not to resuscitate him. His mother insisted he should be, and look at him now. From now on, this will cause serious ethical issues over whether to let such coma victims die."

Still another testimony to the power of Zolpidem to awaken the brain is Heidi Greven. During birth her brain was starved of oxygen. Reflecting back, her mother, Babs, recounted how her daughter always looked dreadfully unhappy, how she would sit unmoving, never communicating in any way. Since she has been taking the "miracle drug" it is as if she has been reborn. She walks around and exhibits curiosity about everything. Though she tends to be silent around strangers she jokes with her doctor and regularly talks with her parents.

"I'll never forget the first time she was given the medication," Babs reminisces. "It was in July 2002. After 10 to 15 minutes it was like a curtain being lifted from her eyes. I couldn't believe it. She suddenly started looking around and fiddling with magazines. Then she went outside the door and looked into the other rooms in the surgery. She found a portable radio and put it up to her shoulder and began listening to it. Beforehand, she would just sit there doing nothing. That was a Saturday. When she went to [a special] school on the Monday, her teacher sent a note home asking what we had done to make Heidi come alive."

The list of success stories using the common sleeping pill Zolpidem is long. One last example:

In 1998, the car driven by 27 year old George Melendez of Houston, Texas overturned into a garden pond during an accident. George ended up with his face underwater. Unable to breathe his brain was starved of oxygen and he went into a deep coma. Three weeks later his body had multiple organ failures and the doctors told his mother Pat that George was clinically dead, a "vegetable" who would never regain consciousness and that it was only a matter of time before his body had total failure and death.

Four years later, to the surprise of the doctors, George was still alive, albeit in very bad shape. Pat and her husband Del had taken George to visit a clinic. While staying the night in a local hotel, Pat became concerned that George's constant moaning might be keeping her husband awake so she decided to give him a sleeping pill. A grateful Pat describes what followed. "After 10 to 15 minutes I noticed there was no sound and I looked over. Instead of finding him asleep, there he was, wide awake, looking at his surroundings. I said, "George," and he said, "What?" We sat up for two hours asking him questions and he answered all of them. His improvements have continued and we talk every day. He has a terrific sense of humor and he carries on running jokes from the day before.

It is difficult to describe how it feels to get someone back who you were told you had lost forever. There is a bond that has been restored and it validates our absolute belief that all along George was locked inside there somewhere. It tells us that we were right and the doctors were wrong. George and his personality were in there the whole time."

When the results of Louis Viljoen's awakening were published in local newspaper articles in South Africa, they caught the attention of Dr. Ralf Clauss, a nuclear medicine physician. He contacted Dr. Nel and suggested using a radioactive isotope diagnostic scan to see if they could determine how Zolpidem was so dramatically affecting Louis. "The results were so unbelievable that I got other colleagues to check my findings," says Dr. Clauss. "We did scans before and after we gave Louis Zolpidem. Areas that appeared black and dead beforehand began to light up with activity afterwards. I was dumbfounded - and I still am."

Dr. Clauss was astounded to see immediate improvements in the left parietal lobe and the left lentiform nucleus was visible. These are critical areas of the brain for motor function, sight, speech and hearing.

"I remember saying to Dr. Nel that we were witnessing medical history," recalls Dr. Clauss.

It is still somewhat of a mystery how the ingredients in a common sleeping pill can awaken seemingly dead brain cells. But doctors Nel and Clauss have made their own preliminary hypothesis based upon the brain chemical called GABA (gamma amino butyric acid).

When a person's brain suffers severe trauma GABA shuts down brain functions to help the cells survive. In long-term coma patients these areas show up as completely dead and inactive and it has been assumed until Zolpidem proved otherwise that these parts of the brain had become irreversibly dead. But the amazing results with Zolpidem are leading many medical specialists to consider that perhaps the brain has just gone into hibernation.

As more research is conducted with comatose patients, the realization is dawning that during the increase of GABA in the brain inducing a coma, the cells are not only shut down, but also somehow changed, causing them to react completely differently than normal cells to subsequent chemical intervention. When the sleeping pill is administered, instead of causing the patient to be sedated it awakens them and brings back long-lost function that had been erroneously assumed was lost forever.

Professor Mike Sathekge, head of nuclear medicine at Pretoria Academic Hospital and Professor Ben Meyer, a renowned South African physician, have been conducting trials of Zolpidem on 30 patients. Professor Meyer explained the significance of the brain awakenings they were seeing after administering just a single dose of the medication. "The results so far could be potentially very important. We have never before spoken of damaged cells in the brain going into hibernation - we have thought of them as necrotic, or dead, cells. But we know cells can go into hibernation in the heart and thyroid, so why not the brain? If there are hibernating cells in damaged brains, it may be that this drug helps to wake them in some people."

In 2007, 360 patients in long-term vegetative states had been participating in worldwide trials to clinically record the effects of Zolpidem on coma patients. This is a preliminary step to mass production and availability of a drug that shows great promise to also benefit stroke victims and other patients with brain-affected challenges.

So far the results have reinforced all of the earlier results. Amy Pickard is one of the 360 trial patients. She had been in a completely unaware and unresponsive coma since experimenting with heroin 6 years earlier. Like many other patients that have received a dose of Zolpidem, Amy's results have been quick and dramatic. Her mother Thelma Pickard says she never lost hope for recovery and said, the "old sparkle" returned to her daughter's eyes when she was given a pill and described the change as "amazing".

Until she began taking Zolpidem for the clinical trials Amy lay seemingly lifeless in a bed in a nursing home kept alive on machines. Just a little over 4 weeks later she was breathing by herself, reacting to the tastes of food, grimacing with something sour and smiling with something sweet, aware of her surroundings, making many voluntary noises and even stood up with the help of two nurses. Her mother exclaimed, "She is changing and it is amazing. When she takes the pill, I see her face relax and the old sparkle return to her eyes. It's incredible. When I look at her now I can see the old Amy coming through, fighting to get out. It's a day-to-day waiting game to see what will happen next, but I just know she's going to speak any day."

When considering the salient point of the wonderful effects of Zolpidem, it is not that this one drug is the single answer, but that it has forever altered long-held medical assumptions about persistent vegetative states and euthanasia. The door is now open for even more marvelous results as additional therapies and chemicals are tried in treatments and rehabilitation. The Filos Treatment that follows is a natural therapy at the forefront of these new medical miracles.

Chapter VII

THE PHILOS TREATMENT

Philos is a trance-channeled higher being, who speaks through Embrosewyn Tazkuvel of the Celestine Light. He has been sharing his wisdom and insights with the world since 1996 on a wide range of topics. Even if you completely disbelieve in channeled higher beings, please take the time to read the recommendations Philos gives. They may make the difference you have been seeking. Nothing is lost and everything may be gained by reading what he has to say.

How to Awaken Someone from a Coma

By Philos the Galactic

During a coma the brain is in shock. Initially, it is likely that the rest of the body is as well. The brain shuts down to try to preserve itself. Many neuro-receptors cease functioning. Unfortunately, doctors often classify someone in such a state as "a vegetable," and tell the family there is no hope and that even if the person did regain consciousness, they wouldn't have a mind left. However, this is not true in more cases than not.

Once the brain has shut down, it has a great deal of difficulty restarting. But unless there was major physical damage to the brain from an accident or wound, (and in some cases even then), it is still ready to be reignited given the right stimulus. In many cases, it is capable of full recovery without loss of any capabilities or capacity. Unfortunately, many people are taken off life support needlessly when all that was required was a little more patience coupled with the correct nutrition and the proper stimulus.

When the conscious brain shuts down in a coma, the "Night Self" takes over. It appears from the oldest and most primitive parts of the brain. The Night Self is a sentient and aware aspect of each person that most people are very disconnected from in the conscious state. In a non-coma state the Night Self is only active for 4-6 hours each day on average. However, in the case of a person in a coma, the Night Self may be active for all 24 hours of the day. Unless stimuli are present to bring the Day Self, the normal daytime, conscious awake aspect, back to the forefront, it can be lost, and the brain simply loses the ability to restart into the awake and conscious state.

Do you recall times when you were asleep but beginning to awaken and were dimly aware of sounds and activity around you? Often times, if you are still too deep in sleep, your brain will incorporate these sounds into actions in dreams you are having. The same principle works in reverse with a person in a coma. Their Night Self is likely off traveling having a great and glorious time somewhere in the universe, because its awareness, consciousness and mobility are not constrained by the limitations of the physical body's location. However, at times, even when in the deepest of coma-like states, due to a lifetime of habit and timing, the Night Self will subside and open the door for the Day Self to reenter. During these windows of opportunity, stimulus from the pre-coma life, if heard, felt or smelled by the person in the coma, will be incorporated into the dreams they are having at the moment. If the stimulus becomes strong enough and occurs during one of these windows of opportunity, the person can awaken from the coma.

Sometimes a person can awaken entirely on their own, and it is considered a miracle. But even then, it probably occurred at a dormant time for the Night Self and during a Day Self window that was successfully activated because of some stimulus from the life of the Day Self during the moment of opportunity. It can be as simple as a single familiar word such as "Dad," "Mom," or even "football practice," if pertinent to the patient and said at the right time.

Even in the case of "irreparable" physical damage to the brain there should be hope for recovery. Though it may be contrary to accepted medical science, the brain can repair itself from physical damage. This includes not only re-growth of new cells, but also rerouting of tasks. If one part of the brain is irreparably damaged but other parts remain in good condition, the human brain can reroute tasks from the normal location of function to an entirely different area of the brain, one that is not usually associated with that function. The steps outlined below will hasten that healing, rerouting and cell regeneration.

Here are the specific techniques to bring someone out of a coma. They are based upon six completely natural pillars-sunshine, oxygen, water, nutrition, physical stimulation and positive reinforcement.

1. **Be patient.** Be patient. Be patient. It can take months, sometimes years, and occasionally even decades for some people to come out of a coma. Be in for the long haul, committed to love them and help them however long it takes. Let your spirit be uplifted with the knowledge that

the techniques that follow will immensely speed up the process of bringing your loved one back to you in fullness.

2. **Believe that they will come out of the coma** and don't give a bit of credence to anything any person or doctor says to the contrary. Your belief is a great power and a tangible force that physically has influence on the person in a coma. Your belief strengthens and entices the Day Self to return,

3. On the flip side, people who doubt the ability of someone to revive from a coma also have power and influence. Their words and attitude entrench the Night Self. **Anyone who holds that doubt should not be allowed to be present** or around the person in a coma. Even in silence, their disbelief energetically reinforces the bonds of the coma.

4. **Never speak or allow doctors or nurses to speak around the person about their condition.** That reinforces the condition and makes it more difficult to be released from its' grip.

5. Your goal is to **provide everyday stimulus and targeted stimulus.** Think about the things you speak about around the dinner table. Talk about school, work, your friends and families lives, big events in town, scandals, anything that you would normally talk about, particularly if it is something pertinent to the person in a coma, such as their school, a practice they need to get to, etc. If you are religious and studied or prayed together continue to do so. (But in their presence, DON"T pray that they would be relieved of their coma. ***They should NEVER hear, feel or understand from any person that they are in a coma***). Involve the person and ask their

opinion, like "what do you think of that?" If you know them well enough, you should be able to respond to the way they would have answered, such as, "I knew you would feel that way about it."

- Also, take frequent opportunities to **physically manipulate** their hands, arms and legs. Hand and foot massages are excellent.

- **Stimulating the sense of smell** is another key component. This should be accomplished with familiar and favored aromas such as hot apple pie or a favorite aroma-filled food, as well as with essential oils in the room, especially those that would have familiarity to the patient. With essential oils it is best to use something like a light bulb ring to hold and heat the essential oils so they permeate the room, but also can be completely removed after the therapy session. This allows a variety of oils to be introduced during different days, continually stimulating the victims' senses, without one aroma simply remaining in the room and being ignored because of 24 hour familiarity. The human olfactory system has the ability to distinguish thousands of different odors and aromas. The memory of these odors is retained deep in the sub-conscious mind. Some form of highly pleasing familiar smells or aromatherapy with essential oils should be used at varying times every day, during the daylight hours, when the patient is either outside in the sun or in a sun-filled room. Stimulation of the olfactory senses is an astoundingly rapid and direct path to the parts of the brain that interpret and respond to sensory input, and highly activating to essential glands.

6. **Pure water** is important. Keeping your loved one well

hydrated with pure water is vital as the brain and the body both utilize the water to good effect. Avoid any water that comes in plastic bottles. The chemicals from the plastic do contaminate the water and are counterproductive and harmful. Also, avoid giving the victim soft drinks, coffee or any kind of sweetened artificial drink or drink containing a drug like caffeine that will affect the body or brain. Even juice should only be pure and fresh squeezed so it nourishes the body and does not contain substances that further degrade it.

7. **Oxygen** is an important piece of putting the shattered brain puzzle back together. And I do not mean oxygen through the nose with a hose from a tank. It should be fresh air from outside, preferably air that has been energized and warmed by the sun or invigorated by a nearby waterfall. Oxygen is the glue that binds the shattered parts of the brain back together, reuniting them in harmony and function. Unfortunately, most patients are kept in rooms with no natural ventilation. The artificial atmosphere may keep them alive, but it will not help awaken them.

8. **Excellent nutrition is essential**. You will probably need to reorient how you think about food and nutrition. Please do not count on the hospital staff to get this right. They have been schooled in the wrong school when it comes to assimilatable and synergistic nutrition. In order for the body and the brain to recuperate and rebuild they must have ample amounts of vital living nutrients that have not been rendered useless by heating or processing so they deliver essential amino acids and nutrients in the most unprocessed, assimilatable and synergistic form. This precludes eating or drinking nutritionless snacks and beverages as well as drinks or foods that would overly

stimulate or depress the body or brain.

- Drinks including caffeine, sugar or alcohol beverages should never be consumed.

- Meat and meat products should also be avoided. Ocean schooling fish are fine.

- You should adhere to a **raw foods diet** with about 70-80% of the foods and drinks you consume. Learn the proper combinations of foods necessary, such as beans and rice, to produce the most complete proteins.

- With beverages, raw freshly made vegetable juices and pure water should be the sole drinks, other than small quantities of fresh-squeezed fruit juices in the morning 1/2 before any food is consumed.

9. The **Thalamus is a critical part** of the brain that must be stimulated to awaken a victim of a coma. This is especially true the longer someone has been in a coma. If your doctors and medical establishment come to understand this, it will be most helpful in the treatments they prescribe. If this key area of the brain has not been physically damaged, it is imperative to stimulate it. Aromatherapy, as I spoke about earlier is very helpful for this purpose. Solar charging the brain as outlined below will also accomplish this, but any additional means that are harmonious with the proper functioning of other parts of the body are beneficial.

10. The next steps are critical and they involve **active interaction with the sun**. You should have your loved one in a coma physically located in a temperately warm, sunny climate and take them outside to just sit in a comfortable morning or afternoon sunshine for ½ hour to an hour

each day. Expose as much of their skin as possible to the sun's rays. Take this opportunity to **use a natural bristle brush** to dry brush off dry and dead skin cells so their refreshed skin can receive maximum benefit from the sunshine.

11. Now the most important thing you can do: **SOLAR CHARGE THE BRAIN**. This will give many more opportunities for the Day Self to come forward and will reactivate, reconnect, repair and regenerate dormant parts of the brain. The life giving sun is the greatest healer given to man. It is a priceless gift of regeneration given from God to humankind and all life on Earth. At the very least, make sure that every day, your loved one is situated in front of a large window facing the daylight. But it is much better to take them outside. Indoors or outdoors, they should be facing as directly toward the sun as possible, even if it is a cloudy day. At night, leave them alone and let them sleep a normal 8 hour sleep cycle undisturbed. Solar Charging also stimulates and reactivates the Thalamus and vital brain glands. Additionally, it will stimulate the regeneration of damaged brain and glandular cells. If there is physical damage to the brain it will take longer for the awakening to manifest as it takes time for cells to regenerate. In all but the most severe cases awakening will occur in time. Please, for the sake of both you and your loved one, be patient.

12. To most effectively bring a victim out of a coma you must **directly give their brain a SOLAR CHARGE**. This cannot be done by artificial

means but must utilize the living sun. Being able to feel the warmth of the sun on the skin is also important.

a). Once the person's body is physically recovered from the trauma that put them in a coma and their retinas are healthy, take them out where their eyes can face the sun, whenever the sun is present, during the first ½ hour of sunrise or the last ½ hour before sunset.

b). Continue with the entire normal conversational stimulus as previously mentioned.

c). When appropriate, physically manipulate their eyelids if necessary, with your fingers and their arms and feet so that they may Sun Gaze in the following manner. It will be best if this is done with them strapped into a sitting position in a wheelchair with their eyes pointing as directly as possible toward the sun.

1). To Sun Gaze, you must find a spot that faces the cresting or falling sun where you can have their ***bare feet*** upon the ***bare earth***. Turn the palms of the hands so they face the sun. In this way, they will benefit not only from the light of the sun but will also be able to become a Vibronic Gateway; an amplifying conduit for the electromagnetic energies of the sun and the planet. A harmonic dance back and forth through their body will begin and benefit them with each passing wave. In order to achieve this, they must have the skin of their bare feet touching the bare ground of the earth. It can be sand, soil or dried mud, but should not be on rock, gravel, concrete, asphalt or any manufactured product. If no bare earth is available green grass is a lesser but acceptable substitute. They should not have their feet in water or wet grass or ground.

2). The area they are in should be open and expansive such as a beach or open field. It should not be cloistered among trees.

3). The sun gazing begins simply and shortly. Their eyelids should remain closed for the initial several sessions. Advance to increasingly longer times and open eye viewing as you feel they are ready.

4). During the first sun gazing session and for as many thereafter as you feel appropriate, face them toward the sun, with their eyes closed and their head angled so that it is facing as directly into the sun as possible. They should be able to feel the heat of the sun upon their eyelids. During the first 1 hour of sunrise and the last 1 hour before sunset the sun may be viewed as long as an hour with their eyelids closed, though you may want to start them with much shorter times until they are acclimated, especially if you are in a tropical latitude where the sun's rays are stronger.

5. When you feel they are ready, begin holding open their eye lids so they are gazing at the sun or just near its' perimeter for 5 seconds only. Do not make them stare unblinking, but blink their eyes for them every few seconds. If you are in the tropics only do this 1/2 hour after sunrise or 1/2 hour before sunset when the sun is not overly intense. You will have the

quickest success using the sunrise time rather than the sunset time, as the sunrise is followed by the daylight, encouraging the Day Self to return, rather than the sunset, which is followed by the night.

6. Speak to them and let them know what you are doing. Tell them you have discovered this wonderful new technique to reinvigorate their mind and body and you want to share it with them. Speak to them thus:

"Clear your mind of all thoughts. Imbue yourself with an attitude of peace, harmony and surrender to the life-giving force of the sun; the sun that gives life to all things on our planet, including you. Repeat to yourself silently that you accept the healing, regenerating, nourishing energy of the sun into every cell of your body, every fiber of your being. Feel your energy expanding outward and upward from deep inside as it is powered and invigorated by the sun, almost lifting your body off the ground. Feel the energy throughout your body coming alive and spinning with vigor, connecting all parts of your body and energy in beneficial and helpful ways, reconnecting, repairing, restoring, and regenerating.

Your body also needs colors for many essential functions. Within the sun are all the colors of the rainbow. See the colors of the rainbow in the sun. Accept them all and allow your body to use whichever it needs wherever they are needed.

Accept the energy of the sun that is entering your body through your eyes, flowing into your brain and

every cell of your body. Understand that this life-giving energy is doing wonderful things to give you health and life. Your belief destroys the walls that hold you back. Your belief physically unlocks the doors to this solar source of life and regeneration. Your belief is your reality. Your belief is your reality. Believe." This is very important.

7. Increase the time they Sun Gaze each day by about 10 seconds. After about 30 sessions, they should be Sun Gazing with open eyes at or about the perimeter of the sun, for about 5 minutes. At this time, all of their tensions, mental distress and anxieties will lessen.

8. Continue for a total of 120 sessions, increasing the gazing time by 10 seconds each day. By the last session, they should be Sun Gazing with open eyes for about 20 minutes each day. (Remember to blink their eyes) They may have already come out of their coma. By the end of the sessions most of their physical ailments and maladies should have disappeared and they should be ready to come out of the coma if they haven't already.

9. There is no need to continue Sun Gazing past the 120th session. After this time, the pineal gland (which is a photosensitive organ with photoreceptor cells, as is the retina), becomes fully activated and the hypothalamus, the pathway from the eye to the brain becomes fully open.

10. The brain and every cell of their body will have become charged with solar energy, the master energy of the planet Earth. They are alive, repairing damage and regenerating! Once their body's cells are thus energized there will no longer be a need to Sun Gaze.

To maintain the cellular charging gained by the Sun Gazing simply put their bare feet 45 minutes each day upon the bare ground facing the sun. It is not necessary to sun gaze with open eyes at this time, but doing so with closed eyelids still gives additional benefits.

11. Continue the stimuli mentioned above at the proper times and daily recharging with bare feet upon bare earth, while facing the sun. In many instances, your loved one will come out of the coma, perfectly normal or will quickly regain their normal state after a few days or weeks of reorientation of their senses and memories.

Go in your light with love & joy,

Philos

APPENDIX

For more information on Sun Gazing please visit the site of the world's Sun Gazing pioneer Hira Ratan Manek, *http://solarhealing.com*

For books by Embrosewyn Tazkuvel please review the front section of the book.

For more information about Celestine Light please visit ***www.celestinelight.org***

OTHER CAPTIVATING, THOUGHT-PROVOKING BOOKS BY

EMBROSEWYN

CELESTINE LIGHT MAGICKAL SIGILS OF HEAVEN AND EARTH

What would happen if you could call upon the blessings of angels and amplify their miracles with the pure essence of spiritual magick?

Miracles manifest! That is the exciting reality that awaits you in *Celestine Light Magickal Sigils of Heaven and Earth.*

Calling upon the higher realm power of angels, through intentional summoning using specific magickal sigils and incantations, is considered to be the most powerful magick of all. But there is a magickal method even greater. When you combine calling upon a mighty angel with adding synergistic sigils and words of power, the amplification of the magickal energy can be astounding and the results that are manifested truly miraculous. This higher technique of magick is the essence of *Celestine Light Magickal Sigils of Heaven and Earth.*

This is the third book of the Magickal Celestine Light series and is an intermediate level reference book for students and practitioners of Celestine Light Magick. It contains a melding of the sigils and names of 99 of the 144 Angels found in *Angels of Miracles and Manifestation*, coupled with synergistic sigils and magickal incantations found within *Words of Power and Transformation*. To fully be able to implement the potent combination of angel magick and words of power magick revealed in this book, the practitioner should have previously read and have available as references the earlier two books in the series.

When magickal incantations and their sigils are evoked in conjunction with the summoning of an angel for a focused purpose, the magickal results are often exceptional. The potent combination of calling upon angels and amplifying your intent with words of power and sigils of spiritual magick creates an awesome, higher magickal energy that can manifest everyday miracles. Employing this potent form of magick can convert challenges into opportunities, powerfully counter all forms of negative magick, entities, phobias, fears and people, greatly enhance good fortune, and help change ordinary lives into the extraordinary.

ANGELS OF MIRACLES AND MANIFESTATION
144 Names, Sigils and Stewardships To Call the Magickal Angels of Celestine Light

You are not alone. Whatever obstacle or challenge you face, whatever threat or adversary looms before you, whatever ability you seek to gain or mountain of life you want to conquer, divine angelic help is ready to intervene on your behalf. When the unlimited power of magickal angels stand with you, obstacles become opportunities, low times become springboards for better days, relationships blossom, illness becomes wellness, challenges become victories and miracles happen!

In *Angels of Miracles and Manifestation*, best-selling spiritual, magickal and paranormal author Embrosewyn Tazkuvel, reveals the secrets to summoning true magickal angels. And once called, how to use their awesome divine power to transform your compelling needs and desires into manifested reality.

Angel magick is the oldest, most powerful and least understood of all methods of magick. Ancient books of scripture from multiple religions tell of the marvelous power and miracles of angels. But the secrets of the true angel names, who they really are, their hierarchy, their stewardship responsibilities, their sigils, and how to successfully call them and have them work their divine magick for you, was lost to the world as a large part of it descended into the dark ages.

But a covenant was made by the Archangel Maeádael to the Adepts of Magick that as the people of the world evolved to a higher light the knowledge and power of angels would come again to the earth during the time of the Generation of Promise. That time is now. We are the Generation of Promise that has been foretold of for millennium. And all that was lost has been restored.

It doesn't matter what religion or path of enlightenment and empowerment that you travel: Wicca, Christianity, Pagan, Jewish, Buddhist, Occult, Muslim, Kabbalah, Vedic, something else or none at all. Nor does your preferred system of magick from Enochian, Thelemic, Gardnerian, Hermetic, to Tantric matter. Once you know the true names of the mighty angels, their unique sigils, and the simple but specific way to summon them, they will come and they will help you.

This revealing book of the ancient Celestine Light magick gives you immediate access to the divine powers of 14 Archangels, 136 Stewardship Angels, and hundreds of Specialty Angels that serve beneath them. Whether you are a novice or a magickal Adept you will find that when angels are on your side you manifest results that you never imagined possible except in your dreams.

The angel magick of Celestine Light is simple and direct without a lot of ritual, which makes it easy even for the novice to be able to quickly use it and gain benefit. While there is a place and importance to ritual in other types of magickal conjuring it is not necessary with angels. They are supernatural beings of unlimited power and awareness whose stewardship includes responding quickly to people in need who call upon them. You do not need elaborate rituals to get their attention.

If you are ready to have magick come alive in your life; if you are ready for real-life practical results that bring wisdom, happiness, health, love and abundance; if you are ready to unveil your life's purpose and unleash your own great potential, obtain the treasure that is this book. Call upon the magickal angels and they will come. But be prepared. When you summon angels, the magick happens and it is transformative. Your life will improve in ways big and small. But it will never be the same.

Want to know more? Take a moment to click on the Look Inside tab in the upper left of this page to see the full extent of the marvels that await you inside this book!

WORDS OF POWER AND TRANSFORMATION
101+ Magickal Words and Sigils of Celestine Light To Manifest Your Desires

Whatever you seek to achieve or change in your life, big or small, Celestine Light magickal words and sigils can help your sincere desires become reality.

Drawing from an ancient well of magickal power, the same divine source used by acclaimed sorcerers, witches and spiritual masters through the ages, the 101+ magickal words and sigils are revealed to the public for the very first time. They can create quick and often profound improvements in your life.

It doesn't matter what religion you follow or what you believe or do not believe. The magickal words and sigils are like mystical keys that open secret doors regardless of who holds the key. If you put the key in and turn it, the door will open and the magick will swirl around you!

From the beginner to the Adept, the Celestine Light words of power and sigils will expand your world and open up possibilities that may have seemed previously unachievable. Everything from something simple like finding a lost object, to something powerful like repelling a psychic or physical attack, to something of need such as greater income, to something life changing like finding your Soul Mate.

Some may wonder how a few spoken words combined with looking for just a moment at a peculiar image could have such immediate and often profound effects. The secret is these are ancient magick words of compelling power and the sigils are the embodiment of their magickal essence. Speaking or even thinking the words, or looking at or even picturing the sigil in your mind, rapidly draws angelic and magickal energies to you like iron to a magnet to fulfill the worthy purpose you desire.

This is a book of potent white magick of the light. Without a lot of training or ritual, it gives you the ability to overcome darkness threatening you from inside or out. For what is darkness except absence of the light? When light shines, darkness fades and disappears, not with a roar, but with a whimper.

Use the words and sigils to call in the magickal energies to transform and improve your life in every aspect. In this comprehensive book you will find activators to propel your personal growth, help you excel in school, succeed in your own business, or launch you to new heights in your profession. It will give you fast acting keys to improve your relationships, change your luck, revitalize your health, and develop and expand your psychic abilities.

Embrosewyn Tazkuvel is an Adept of the highest order in Celestine Light. After six decades of using magick and teaching it to others he is now sharing some of the secrets of what he knows with you. Knowledge that will instantly connect you to divine and powerful universal forces that with harmonic resonance, will unleash the magickal you!

Inside you will discover:

- 101 word combinations that call in magickal forces like a whirlwind of light.

- 177 magickal words in total.

- 101 sigils to go with each magickal word combination to amplify the magickal results you seek.

- 101 audio files you can listen to; helping you have perfect pronunciation of the Words of Power regardless of your native language. Available directly from the eBook and with a link in the paperback edition.

AURAS
How To See, Feel & Know

***Auras: How to See, Feel & Know*, is like three books in one!**

1. It's an information packed, full color, complete training manual with 17 time tested exercises and 47 photos and illustrations to help you quickly be able to see Auras in vibrant color! It is the only full color book on auras available.

2. An entertaining read as Embrosewyn recalls his early childhood and high school experiences seeing auras, and the often humorous reactions by everyone from his mother to his friends when he told them what he saw.

3. Plus, a fascinating chapter on body language. Embrosewyn teaches in his workshops to not just rely on your interpretation of the aura alone, but to confirm it with another indicator such as body language.*Auras: How to See, Feel & Know*, goes in depth with thorough explanations and great pictures to show you all the common body language indicators used to confirm what someone's aura is showing you.

Auras includes:

- 17 dynamic eye exercises to help you rapidly begin to see the beautiful world of auras!
- 47 full color pictures and illustrations (in the Kindle or Full Color print edition).

Anyone with vision in both eyes can begin seeing vividly colored auras around any person with just 5 minutes of practice!

Learn how to:

- See the 7 layers of the aura using Embrosewyn's pioneering technique
- Understand the meaning of the patterns and shadows observed in the layers
- Train your eyes to instantly switch back and forth from aura to normal vision
- Understand the meaning and nuances of every color of the rainbow in an aura
- Use your aura as a shield against negative energy or people
- Power up your aura to have greater achievement in any endeavor
- Interpret body language to confirm observations of the aura
- Cut negative energy cords to disharmonious people
- Understand health conditions and ailments through the aura

The secret to aura sight is to retrain the focusing parts of your eyes to see things that have always been there, but you have never been able to see before. It's really not complicated. Anyone can do it using Embrosewyn's proven techniques and eye exercises. The author has been seeing brightly colored auras for over 60 years and teaching others to begin seeing auras within 5 minutes for the last 22 years. *Auras: How to See, Feel & Know*, includes all the power techniques, tools and Full Color eye exercises from his popular workshops.

For those who already have experience seeing auras, the deeper auric layers and subtle auric nuances and the special ways to focus your eyes to see them, are explained in detail, with Full Color pictures andillustrations to show you how the deeper layers and auric aberrations appear. It is also a complete training manual to help you quickly be able to see Auras in vibrant color. It includes 17 eye exercises and dozens of Full Color pictures, enabling anyone with vision in both eyes to begin seeing vividly colored auras around any person. The secret is in retraining the focusing parts of your eyes to see things that have always been there, but you have never been able to see before. *Auras: How to See, Feel & Know*, includes all the power techniques, tools and Full Color eye exercises from Embrosewyn's popular workshops.

Additionally, there is a fascinating chapter on body language. Embrosewyn teaches in his workshops to not just rely on your interpretation of the aura alone, but to confirm it with another indicator such as body language. *Auras: How to See, Feel & Know* goes in depth with thorough explanations and great pictures to show you all the common body language indicators used to confirm what someone's aura is showing you.

For those who already have experience seeing auras, the deeper auric layers and subtle auric nuances and the special ways to focus your eyes to see them, are explained in detail, with accompanying Full Color pictures to show you how the deeper layers and auric aberrations appear.

SOUL MATE AURAS
How to Find Your Soul Mate & "Happily Ever After"

Find your own "Happily Ever After."

Experience the joy of finding your Soul Mate. Learn the simple secrets to discovering the love of your life!

Soul Mate Auras: How to Find Your Soul Mate & "Happily Ever After" uses dozens of full color pictures and the experience of 60 years of seeing auras, to give you the master keys to unlock the passageway to discovering your Soul Mate using the certainty of your auric connections. Every person has a unique aura and auric field generated by their seven energy centers. Find the person that you resonate strongly with on all seven energy centers and you'll find your Soul Mate!

You can sense and see auras, even if you never have!

In *Soul Mate Auras* full color eye and energy exercises will help you learn how to see and feel auras and how to use that ability to identify where in the great big world your Soul Mate is living. Once you are physically in the presence of your prospective Soul Mate, you will know how to use your aura to energetically confirm that they are the one. The same methods can be used to discover multiple people that are Twin Flames with you; not quite seven auric connection Soul Mates, but still deep and expansive connections to you on five to six energy centers.

Soul Mate Auras also includes an in-depth checklist method to determine if someone is your Twin Flame or Soul Mate.

This is a proven method of confirmation, not by using your aura, but by honestly and rationally evaluating your connections on all seven of your energy centers. This is an invaluable tool for anyone contemplating marriage or entering into a long-term committed relationship. It also serves as a useful second opinion confirmation for anyone that has used their aura to find their Soul Mate.

To help inspire and motivate you to create your own "happily ever after," Soul Mate Auras is richly accentuated with dozens of full color photos of loving couples along with profound quotes from famous to anonymous people about the wonder of Soul Mates.

Treat yourself to the reality of finding your Soul Mate or confirming the one that you have already found!

Secret Earth Series

INCEPTION
BOOK 1

Could it be possible that there is a man alive on the Earth today that has been here for two thousand years? How has he lived so long? And why? What secrets does he know? Can his knowledge save the Earth or is it doomed?

Continuing the epic historical saga begun in the *Oracles of Celestine Light*, but written as a novel rather than a chronicle, *Inception* unveils the life and adventures of Lazarus of Bethany and his powerful and mysterious sister Miriam of Magdala.

The first book of the Secret Earth series, *Inception*, reveals the hidden beginnings of the strange, secret life of Lazarus. From his comfortable position as the master of caravans to Egypt he is swept into a web of intrigue involving his enigmatic sister Miriam and a myriad of challenging dangers that never seem to end and spans both space and time.

Some say Miriam is an angel, while others are vehement that she is a witch. Lazarus learns the improbable truth about his sister, and along with twenty-three other courageous men and women, is endowed with the secrets of immortality. But he learns that living the secrets is not as easy as knowing them. And living them comes at a price; one that needs to be paid in unwavering courage, stained with blood, built with toil, and endured with millenniums of sacrifice, defending the Earth from all the horrors that might have been. *Inception* is just the beginning of their odyssey.

DESTINY
BOOK 2

In preparation, before beginning their training as immortal Guardians of the Earth, Lazarus of Bethany and his wife Hannah were asked to go on a short visit to a world in another dimension. "Just to look around a bit and get a feel for the differences," Lazarus's mysterious sister, Miriam of Magdala assured them.

She neglected to mention the ravenous monstrous birds, the ferocious fire-breathing dragons, the impossibly perfect people with sinister ulterior motives, and the fact that they would end up being naked almost all the time! And that was just the beginning of the challenges!

UNLEASH YOUR PSYCHIC POWERS

A Comprehensive 400 Page Guidebook

Unleash Your Psychic Powers is an entertaining, enlightening and educational resource for all levels of practitioners in the psychic, magickal and paranormal arts. It includes easy-to-follow, step-by-step instructions on how you can develop and enhance the full potential of dynamic psychic, magickal and paranormal powers in your own life.

Whether You Are A Novice Or An Adept

You will find valuable insight and guidance, based upon Embrosewyn's six decades of experience discovering and developing psychic and paranormal talents and unleashing the power of the magickal arts.

Twenty Psychic And Paranormal Abilities Are Explored

Including well known abilities such as Clairvoyance, Telekinesis, Telepathy, Lucid Dreaming, Precognition, Astral Projection and Faith Healing, plus, more obscure talents such as Channeling, Dowsing, and Automatic Handwriting.

In addition to helping you develop and master the psychic abilities that call to you, each of the twenty powers described are spiced with fascinating personal stories from the lives of Embrosewyn and others, to help you understand some of the real world consequences and benefits of using these formidable magickal and psychic talents. Paranormal abilities have saved Embrosewyn's life and the lives of his family members on multiple occasions. Learning to fully develop your own psychic and paranormal abilities may come in just as handy one day.

For anyone that is an active spirit medium, or uses any psychic abilities involving other-worldly beings, such as divination, channeling, or ghost hunting, the chapter on

Psychic Self-defense is an extensive must read, covering low, medium and high risk threats, including everything from negative vortexes, to entities, energy vampires, ghosts, aliens and demons. Exorcism, and how to protect both people and property from unseen forces is also completely explained.

Filled with pictures and vivid descriptions of how you can bring forth and develop your own transcendental supernatural gifts, *Unleash Your Psychic Powers* should be in the library of every serious student of the psychic, magickal, paranormal and supernatural.

Everyone has psychic and paranormal abilities. It is your birthright! You were born with them!

Within this book you'll learn how to unlock and unleash your astounding supernatural potential and the amazing things you can do with your powers once they are free!

PSYCHIC SELF DEFENSE

A Complete Guide to Protecting Yourself Against Psychic & Paranormal Attack (and just plain irksome people)

Felt a negative energy come over you for no apparent reason when you are near someone or around certain places? Had a curse hurled at you? Spooked by a ghost in a building? Imperiled by demonic forces? Being drained and discombobulated by an energy vampire? Or, do you encounter more mundane but still disruptive negative energies like an over demanding boss, the local bully, hurtful gossip, a physically or mentally abusive spouse, or life in a dangerous neighborhood threatened by thieves and violence? Whatever your source of negative energy, danger or threat, you'll find effective, proven, psychic and magickal countermeasures within this book.

Psychic Self Defense draws upon Embrosewyn's six decades of personal experience using psychic abilities and magickal defenses to thwart, counter and send back to sender, any and all hostile paranormal threats. Everything from unsupportive and dismissive family and friends, to ghosts, demons and exorcisms. The same practical and easy to learn Magickal techniques can be mastered by anyone serious enough to give it some time and practice, and can aid you immensely with a host of material world challenges as well.

17 psychic and paranormal threats are covered with exact, effective counter measures, including many real life examples from Embrosewyn's comprehensive personal experiences with the paranormal, devising what works and what doesn't from hard won trial and error.

Whether you are a medium needing to keep foul spirits

away, or simply someone desiring to know that you, your family and property are safe and protected, you will find the means to insure peace and security with the proven methods outlined in *Psychic Self Defense*

You will learn how to:

- Create your own Magick spells tailored to your particular situation and need
- Call upon specific angels to aid you
- Create Crystal Energy Shields
- Protect yourself when in a channeling or spirit medium trance
- Use your Aura to create ASP's (Auric Shields of Power)
- Empower Wards for protection against specific threats
- Recognize and counter Energy Vampires
- Cleanse a home of negative energy
- Cut negative energy cords to disharmonious people
- Counter Black Magick
- Detect alien presence
- Banish malicious entities or demons

Though dealing with numerous and sometimes dangerous other-worldly and material world threats, the entire approach of this book is from a position of personal empowerment, no fear, and divine white light. Whether you are religious or an atheist, an experienced practitioner of the psychic and magickal arts or a neophyte, someone living in a haunted house or just an employee wanting to have a nicer boss, there will be hundreds of ways you can use the information in this book to help you in your life. And you will learn to do it in ways that are uplifting and empowering, producing results that are peaceful, safe and harmonious.

Psychic Self Defense is also available as an AUDIO BOOK.

22 STEPS TO THE LIGHT OF YOUR SOUL

A Treasured Book That Will Help You Unleash The Greatness Within

What would it be like if you could reach through space and time to query the accumulated wisdom of the ages and get an answer? *22 Steps to the Light of Your Soul* reveals such treasured insights, eloquently expounding upon the foundational principles of 22 timeless subjects of universal interest and appeal, to help each reader grow and expand into their fullest potential.

In a thought-provoking, poetic writing style, answers to questions we all ponder upon, such as love, happiness, success and friendship, are explored and illuminated in short, concise chapters, perfect for a thought to ponder through the day or contemplate as your eyes close for sleep.

Each paragraph tells a story and virtually every sentence could stand alone as an inspiring quote on your wall.

These are the 22 steps of the Light of Your Soul

Step 1: The Purpose of Life
Step 2: Balance
Step 3: Character
Step 4: Habits
Step 5: Friendship
Step 6: True Love
Step 7: Marriage
Step 8: Children
Step 9: Happiness
Step 10: Play & Relaxation
Step 11: Health

Step 12: Success
Step 13: Knowledge
Step 14: Passion & Serenity
Step 15: Imagination & Vision
Step 16: Creativity & Art
Step 17: Adversity
Step 18: Respect
Step 19: Freedom & Responsibility
Step 20: Stewardship
Step 21: Faith
Step 22: Love Yourself - the Alpha and the Omega

ALSO AVAILABLE AS AN AUDIO BOOK! You can listen as you commute to work or travel on vacation, or even listen and read together!

LOVE YOURSELF
The Secret Key to Transforming Your Life

Loving yourself is all about energy

As humans we devote a great deal of our energy through our time, thoughts and emotions to love. We read about it, watch movies and shows about it, dream about it, hope for it to bless our lives, feel like something critically important is lacking when it doesn't, and at the very least keep a sharp eye out for it when its missing.

Too often we look to someone else to fulfill our love and crash and burn when relationships end, or fail to live up to our fantasies of what we thought they should be. When we seek love from another person or source greater than the love we give to ourselves, we set ourselves up to an inevitable hard landing when the other person or source ceases to provide the level of fulfillment we desire.

Loving yourself is a precious gift from you to you. It is an incredibly powerful energy that not only enhances your ability to give love more fully to others, it also creates a positive energy of expanding reverberation that brings more love, friendship and appreciation to you from all directions. It is the inner light that illuminates your life empowering you to create the kind of life you desire and dream.

The relationship you have with yourself is the most important one in your life. Happiness will forever be fleeting if you do not have peace, respect and love for yourself. It's not selfish. It's not vain. It is in fact the key to transforming your life. Inward reflection and appreciation will open up clearer channels to the divine. Relationships with everyone will be enhanced as your relationship with yourself expands and is uplifted.

All other relationships are only mirrors of the one you

have within. As you love yourself, are kind to yourself, respect yourself, so too will you be able to give those and so many other good qualities to others in equal measure to that which you give to yourself.

This is a short, but very sweet book to help you discover your inner glow of love. Within its covers are two great keys you will find no other place. These two keys will proactively bring you to the serenity of self-love regardless of whether you are currently near or far from that place of peace.

Are you familiar with the infinity symbol? It looks pretty much like the number 8 turned on its side. As love for yourself should be now and forever, in the last chapter you will find 88 reasons why loving yourself is vitally important to your joy, personal growth and expansion, and the happiness of everyone whose lives you touch. Most people have never considered that there could be a list that long just about loving yourself! But with each short phrase you read your mind begins to understand to a greater depth how important loving yourself is for all aspects of your life and relationships. As your mind understands your life follows.

This book leaves you with a special gift Inside you'll find two short, but very valuable multimedia flash presentations. One is entitled "Forgive Yourself". The other is "Love Yourself" These are not normal flash presentations. They are self-hypnosis, positive affirmations that will rapidly help you achieve greater self-love and more fulfilling love-filled realities in your life. As soft repetitive music plays in the background, images reinforcing the theme will flash by on your screen about three per second, accompanied by short phrases superimposed on a portion of the image. In a quick 7-10 minute session, sitting at home in front of your computer, you will find the flash presentations buoy and motivate you. Repeat them twice a day for several days and you will find they are transformative.

Special Bonus: *Love Yourself* is ALSO AVAILABLE AS

AN AUDIO BOOK! This allows you to listen and read at the same time!

ORACLES OF CELESTINE LIGHT
Complete Trilogy Of Genesis, Nexus & Vivus

Once in a lifetime comes a book that can dramatically change your life for the better - forever. This is it!

WHAT WAS LOST...HAS BEEN FOUND

This is the complete 808 page trilogy of the Celestine books of Light: Genesis, Nexus and Vivus.

The controversial *Oracles of Celestine Light*, is a portal in time to the days of Yeshua of Nazareth, over 2000 years ago, revealed in fulfilling detail to the world by the reclusive Embrosewyn Tazkuvel. It includes 155 chapters of sacred wisdom, miracles and mysteries revealing life-changing knowledge about health, longevity, happiness and spiritual expansion that reverberates into your life today.

Learn the startling, never before understood truth:

About aliens, other dimensions, Atlantis, Adam & Eve, the Garden of Eden, Noah and the ark, giants, the empowerment of women, dreams, angels, Yeshua of Nazareth (Jesus), his crucifixion & resurrection, his wife Miriam of Magdala (Mary Magdala), Yudas Iscariot (Judas), the afterlife, reincarnation, energy vortexes, witches, magic, miracles, paranormal abilities, and you!

The **Or***acles of Celestine Light* turns accepted religious history and traditional teachings on their head. But page by page, it makes more sense than anything you´ve ever read and shares simple yet profound truths to make your life better today and help you to understand and unleash your miraculous potential.

The *Oracles of Celestine Light* explains who you are, why you are here, and your divine destiny. It is a must-read for anyone interested in spirituality, personal growth and thought-provoking answers to the unknown.

"You are a child of God, a Child of Light, literally a priceless son or daughter of divinity. Even through the fog of mortal upheavals and the tumults and tribulations, always remember you are still a child of God and shall inherit joy and kingdoms beyond measure, as you remain true to your light."

Genesis 11:99

Psychic Awakening Series

CLAIRVOYANCE

Would it be helpful if you could gain hidden knowledge about a person, place, thing, event, or concept, not by any of your five physical senses, but with visions and "knowing?"

Are you ready to supercharge your intuition? *Clairvoyance* takes you on a quest of self-discovery and personal empowerment, helping you unlock this potent ESP ability in your life. It includes riveting stories from Embrosewyn's six decades of psychic and paranormal adventures, plus fascinating accounts of others as they discovered and cultivated their supernatural abilities.

Clearly written, step-by-step practice exercises will help you to expand and benefit from your own psychic and clairvoyant abilities. This can make a HUGE improvement in your relationships, career and creativity. As Embrosewyn has proven from over twenty years helping thousands of students to find and develop their psychic and paranormal abilities, EVERYONE, has one or more supernatural gifts. *Clairvoyance* will help you discover and unleash yours!

If you are interested in helping yourself to achieve more happiness, better health, greater knowledge, increased wealth and a deeper spirituality, unlocking your power of clairvoyance can be the key. Hidden knowledge revealed becomes paths unseen unveiled.

Unleashing your psychic gifts does more than just give you advantage in life challenges. It is a safe, ethical, even spiritual and essential part of you that makes you whole, once you accept that you have these special psychic abilities and begin to use them.

TELEKINESIS

Easy, comprehensive guide for anyone wanting to develop the supernatural ability of Telekinesis

Telekinesis, also known as psychokinesis, is the ability to move or influence the properties of objects without physical contact. Typically it is ascribed as a power of the mind. But as Embrosewyn explains, based upon his sixty years of personal experience, the actual physical force that moves and influences objects emanates from a person's auric field. It initiates with a mental thought, but the secret to the power is in your aura!

Telekinesis is the second book in the Psychic Awakening series by popular paranormal writer Embrosewyn Tazkuvel. The series was specifically created to offer short, inexpensive, information filled handbooks to help you quickly learn and develop specific psychic and paranormal abilities.

Clearly written, *Telekinesis* is filled with step-by-step practice exercises and training techniques proven to help you unlock this formidable paranormal ability. Spiced with riveting accounts of real-life psychic experiences and paranormal adventures, you'll be entertained while you learn. But along the way you will begin to unleash the potent power of Telekinesis in your own life!

As Embrosewyn has proven from over twenty years helping thousands of students to find and develop their psychic and paranormal abilities. EVERYONE, has one or more supernatural gifts. Is Telekinesis one of yours? Perhaps it's time to find out.

DREAMS

Awaken in the world of your sleep

In *Dreams*, the third book of the Psychic awakening series, renowned psychic/paranormal practitioner Embrosewyn Tazkuvel reveals some of his personal experiences with the transformational effect of dreams, while sharing time-tested techniques and insights that will help you unlock the power of your own night travels.

Lucid Dreaming

An expanded section on Lucid Dreaming gives you proven methods to induce and develop your innate ability to control your dreams. It explores the astonishing hidden world of your dream state that can reveal higher knowledge, greatly boost your creativity, improve your memory, and help you solve vexing problems of everyday life that previously seemed to have no solution.

Nine Types of Dreams

Detailing the nine types of dreams will help you to understand which dreams are irrelevant and which you should pay close attention to, especially when they reoccur. You'll gain insight into how to interpret the various types of dreams to understand which are warnings and which are gems of inspiration that can change your life from the moment you awaken and begin to act upon that which you dreamed.

Become the master of your dreams

Sleeping and dreaming are a part of your daily life that cumulatively accounts for dozens of years of your total life. It is a valuable time of far more than just rest. Become the master of your dreams and your entire life can become more than you ever imagined possible. Your dreams are the secret key to your future.

Additional Services Offered by Embrosewyn

~ on a limited basis ~

I am honored to be able to be of further service to you by offering multiple paranormal abilities for your enlightenment and life assistance. On a limited basis as my time allows I can: discover your Soul Name and the meaning and powers of the sounds; custom craft and imbue enchantments upon a piece of your jewelry for a wide beneficial range of purposes; discover the name of your Guardian Angel; have an in-depth psychic consultation and Insight Card reading with you via a Skype video call. My wife Sumara can also create a beautiful piece of collage art on 20"x30" internally framed canvas, representing all of the meanings and powers of the sounds of your Soul Name.

If you are interested in learning more about any of these additional services please visit my website, *www.embrosewyn.com* and click on the link at the top for SERVICES.

CPSIA information can be obtained
at www.ICGtesting.com
Printed in the USA
LVHW081604310120
645468LV00032B/1052

9 780938 001058